# HOW TO DEVELOP A POWERFUL GRIP

By

## EDWARD ASTON

# HOW TO DEVELOP A POWERFUL GRIP

(ORIGINAL VERSION, RESTORED)

By

## EDWARD ASTON

Originally published in 1937

PUBLISHED BY O'Faolain Patriot L L C, Copyright 2011

info@PhysicalCultureBooks.com

ISBN-13: 978-1467977845

ISBN-10: 1467977845

Published in the United States of America

To Order More Copies Visit: Physical Culture Books.com

# HOW TO DEVELOP A POWERFUL GRIP

## INTRODUCTION

Everyone of us today should be interested in the possession of a powerful grip. And when I say everyone, I mean everyone: man, woman, boy or girl. For the past six years the British nation has been organised for war on a scale unknown to history, with a roll-call of twenty-three and a half millions enlisted in, or working for, the Services out of a total population of forty-two millions; thus representing the greatest national effort among the Allies. This colossal number was engaged in the Army, Navy, Air ˣForce, Merchant Navy, Civil Defence services or on Munitions, many of them having to make full use of their physical powers—and this applies to both sexes— for the first time in their lives.

No matter whether you were a soldier, sailor, airman, policeman, fireman, air-raid warden or rescue worker, you will agree that the possession of a powerful grip was one of your best physical assets and most of us who served in any of the above capacities are more than grateful because of the service it rendered to us and others. On the other hand, if you were a member of the Land Army, any of the Women's Services, employed on a gun site or a balloon post; or in a munition factory, then you must have experienced occasions when you wished you had more power in your hands; when you fumed at your helplessness at having to wait for the mere male with his superior strength to get you out of your temporary trouble. In those days of enemy action every man or woman could be called upon at any hour of the day or night to use the power of their hands in the work of fire-fighting or rescue after an air raid. In the field, in the air, on board ship, in the mines, in the factory or even in the streets the possession of a pair of strong arms may have saved your own life or that of your fellow man.

Never in the history of our nation was physical fitness so vital to the survival of the race, for every ounce of energy created and utilised in these days of re-habilitation will bring the conquest of peace conditions nearer and this necessary vitality can be created by one method alone: that of physical exercise. Strength creates confidence, the will to do and dare, the energy and initiative to achieve, to lead where others follow, and most important of all: to carry on when all others have given up. And right behind all this is the exultant confidence in one's strong right arm that is the main characteristic of the British bull-dog tenacity to hang on.

Now the greatest factor for the creation of a powerful grip is SHEER WILL POWER, for one cannot develop a more-than-average strength concentrated in the hands and forearms without one possesses the necessary mental force capable of creating and exerting that power. The man with good gripping powers is invariably a man with a mind of his own, knowing what he requires from life and determined to get it. Hundreds of books have been written on the subject of Will Power, extolling the benefits to be derived from the improvement of this mental trait, while the methods to be used in its creation have been variously prescribed from gazing fixedly at a glass crystal to the act of bending down to touch one's toes fifty times every morning, but so far as I can remember not one book has advocated the cultivation of the gripping powers of the hand as a means of strengthening one's character and determination.

Yet we see and hear the connection every day of our lives. A powerful orator is stated to have an excellent grip of his subject and must be able to grip the attention of his audience in order to subordinate their will to his own. The successful student must get a grip of the matter in his text book before he is able to master the subject. The popular author grips the attention of his readers with such power that they have difficulty in closing the book before they have reached the last chapter, no matter what other urgent calls there may be on their time. The prosperous salesman, with his knowledge of practical psychology, must interest his prospective customer in the product, that is to say he must grip his attention before he can create the desire to purchase and so it goes on all through the day, the successful man—and we all have something to sell, if it is only our personality to our friends—must possess "grip."

Have you ever stood by ashamed of your weakness while stronger men have been able to do the things you would have liked to have done? Perhaps you remember a time when you had to keep in the background and let others come forward to do a real man's job, not for lack of grit or courage, but because you realised that you did not possess the necessary muscle power to back that courage and you were afraid of the ridicule to which you might expose yourself if you attempted to take a hand? You feared, not the danger, but the possibility of jibes. You strongly desired the cheers and approbation of the crowd but anticipated their derision as you realised how puny your attempts would appear.

This occasion may arise again today or tomorrow, for who can foretell what is in store for us in these stirring times. So prepare now to meet that situation by so training your body that you will look forward to adventure with courage and determination, instead of fear and doubt. To strengthen the wrist and forearm you need no elaborate equipment, for the hands are always in use and consequently the power of grip is very easy to cultivate. No matter where you are, if you have the will to persevere, any article in everyday use will serve for the purpose of developing your grip.

The man in the Services may be apt to imagine that he gets enough work in his daily training to exercise his powers to the full, but a little reflection should convince him that the stronger he becomes the more efficient a soldier, sailor or airman he will make of himself; the better his prospects of promotion and the greater his chance of survival in battle. The policeman, fire-fighter, etc., may feel that he has had enough of it after his spell of duty is finished, but by keeping himself fighting fit, he will undoubtedly possess reserves of strength to cope with any emergency that may arise. Again, the miner, engineer, labourer or even the black-coat worker will work with greater ease and enjoy their recreation more if they take a greater interest in their physical condition.

To exert your gripping powers you have to bring your mental powers into play. You may perform free exercises until the cows come home with little benefit to your health, strength or muscularity if your mind is wandering from the thoughts of breakfast to your best girl, for it is only when you focus your full attention to the muscles being used that the work becomes strenuous and result-getting. Attempt to pick up a weight from the floor—one just within your compass—and you will find that unless you bring your full powers to bear on the job in hand, you will not succeed in raising it an inch. You have to give your full and undivided attention to the task of raising the weight; otherwise you will fail. We therefore see that the practice of exercises calculated to augment one's gripping powers must of necessity improve and strengthen one's Power of Will with untold benefits to one's whole career.

Now every man, woman or youth would be all the more efficient, both mentally and physically, for the possession of a powerful grip. By this, I do not mean that every woman should go about with her sleeves tucked up displaying a brawny forearm and using her Amazonic strength on all within her reach, for in actual fact a woman does not make a bunchy type of muscle; the feminine muscle being of the long, straited kind, so that it is possible for her to be quite above average in strength and yet possess a smooth, well-rounded arm. Again, a word of warning to the male. The man who grips your fingers so tightly as to crush them and inflict pain on every occasion for a handshake is in all probability suffering from an inverted inferiority complex and must be tolerated until he realises his exertion of physical strength is really a display of mental weakness. Therefore, when you encounter this type, resist the temptation to kick his shins and wait for the next occasion, when by seizing his finger-tips—instead of allowing your whole hand to be engulfed by his palm—you can return the compliment. When you have mastered a few of the exercises that follow, your gripping powers will probably be doubled or tripled in strength, but you in your turn will remember that the strong are the gentle and that the athlete's handshake should be a firm one without undue pressure, creating and imparting a mutual feeling of confidence and friendliness.

Two of the most frequent objections to taking up physical culture that one hears, are, " Oh, Yes, it's a fine thing, but really I simply haven't the time," and "I'm in digs and my landlady would create something awful if I had any gear lying about my room," to both of which the reply is " Objection over-ruled." At least as far as the cultivation of extra strength in the wrist and forearm is concerned, for these parts can be exercised whilst walking to work or waiting for a train or bus, without making oneself in the least conspicuous. Nor need there be any set times for practice—unless one wishes to get into the strong man class—for any odd moments can be utilised for practice. Again, for the average person, there need be no apparatus to purchase and therefore no gear to lumber up your digs. For the housewife, the broom, flat-iron or scrubber will suffice. The manual worker will find opportunities at every moment to improve his grip when handling the tools of his trade. The clerical worker, whose greatest effort during the day may be the handling of a ledger or the manipulation of a fountain pen, can carry his apparatus about with him in the form of a ball of paper—a small india rubber would be better—in his coat pocket and while awaiting his conveyance, he can alternately grip and relax this small object until his wrists ache. An excellent reminder this will be, that he must keep his shoulders square and his chest out; to offset in some small measure his cramped position over the desk.

Now why should the housewife, the manual worker or the clerk worry about their power of grip? Because it will add a little fun to their work, it will so improve their strength that they will get through their work easier, and, strange but true, they will not be wasting energy but increasing it. Instead of being " all out" at the end of the day, they will be ready to enjoy their leisure, for only by using your muscular power, can you create a reserve of muscular energy.

# 1. SQUEEZING A RUBBER BALL.

The squeezing of a rubber ball is excellent practice for the hands and forearms, and will considerably improve the gripping powers of the fingers. Place the ball in the dead centre of the hand and circle it with the fingers, keeping the thumb away. Clench the ball tightly, pressing it against the heel of the thumb and then close ,the thumb on it, turning the wrist inwards slightly. Put some real pressure into the grip and then relax. Continue to grip and relax until the wrist and forearm ache, and then repeat with the other hand. In cold weather a ball may be carried in the overcoat pocket and will provide exercise for the wrists and warmth for the hands.

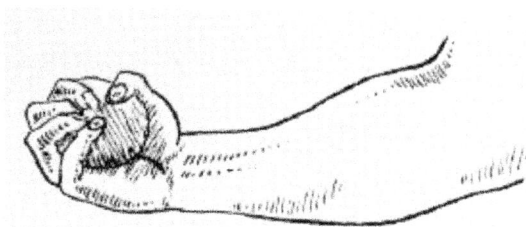

## 2. BREAKING MATCH STICKS WITH THE FINGERS.

This is not so easy as it looks. Place a match stick of full length between the first and third fingers of one hand, just where the finger nails end. (Not on the nails as shewn in the above illustration.) The second or index finger to be on top of the match, between the two fingers. The thumb and little finger are to be kept free so as to render no assistance in breaking the match. Keeping the fingers perfectly straight, the trick is to break the match by pressing down with the second finger and upwards with the first and third. If one is not successful in this position, the feat can be made easier by shifting the match along the fingers towards the hand. Practice with both hands until proficient. Persons with short fingers have an advantage over those with longer digits. Vansittart, " the man with the iron grip," could break the stem of a clay pipe in this manner.

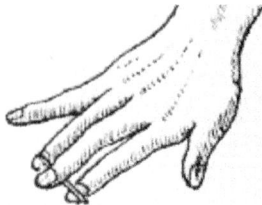

## 3. TWISTING AND TEARING A NEWSPAPER.

After you have finished with your newspapers, do not throw them away as they are needed for salvage. But before parting with them you will be able to get some splendid exercise in this manner. Fold up about six papers to a length of nine or more inches, according to their size, and then roll them up in the form of a cylinder. Commence to twist them by turning inwards with the right hand and outwards with the left, the hands being about three inches apart. Continue until they tear. The feat can be made easier by bringing the hands closer together, as the force is concentrated over a smaller area.

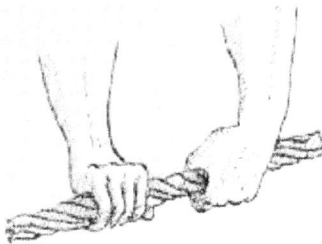

## 4. TURNING JAR TOPS.

Procure a long jar with a screw-on lid. Screw the lid on as tightly as can be managed and then proceed to unscrew it. Hold the bottom of the jar in the left hand and the lid in the right, the fingers of which should be well apart. Now securing a firm grip with both hands turn the left hand to the left and the right hand to the right, when the lid should be eased. If it does not turn at the first attempt, simply keep on until it does, as the action brings into play the whole of the tendons of the hands. As the grip improves the lid can be forced on tighter, with greater benefit in the unscrewing process.

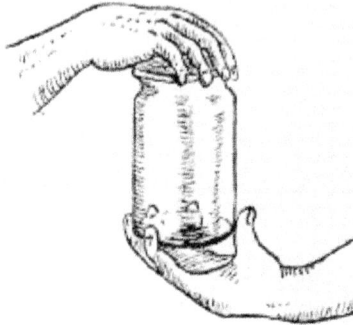

## 5. HOLDING PENNY IN CLOTHES PEG.

This is a simple stunt which will test your endurance more than your actual gripping powers. Procure an ordinary clothes peg and placing a coin between the ends, grip the peg over the penny with the thumb and forefinger sufficiently hard enough to retain the coin in position. The test consists in seeing how long you can retain the coin in the peg without relaxing your grip and you may time yourself with the second hand of a watch. Sixty seconds is a very good try.

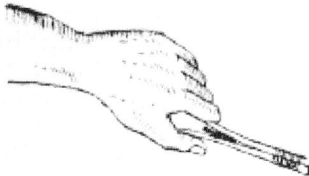

# 6. PICKING UP A CHAIR BY THE LEG.

The correct method of lifting a chair by the leg is to kneel down on the right knee if the right hand is to be used (or the left knee when the left hand is used), the body being at right angles away from the chair so that an advantage of leverage is obtained. The grip should be taken with the fingers up the leg, the little finger being level with the floor. The elbow should also rest on the floor and the chair raised evenly so that all four legs leave the floor at the same time.

If the chair is a heavy one, it will be easier to elevate it by the back leg; although in this case the biceps of the arm will do most of the work instead of the grip. If, even with this added advantage, the feat cannot be accomplished, the hand can be shifted up the leg nearer the seat until it becomes easy. Then, as one's strength improves, the grip can be taken lower and lower until the bottom of the leg can be utilised. After that, the front leg can be tackled.

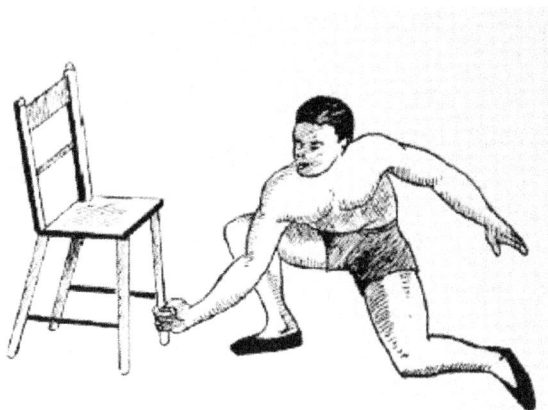

## 7. GRIPPING AN OPEN DOOR.

Here is an exercise that will improve the grip in no time. Practice it in this way. Stand before an open door and with the feet level with the edge, grasp the door at waist height with one hand and bend down until you are sitting on your heels and leaning well back-wards. Practice this with either hand until it becomes easy. Continue by using the thumb and first three fingers only, then thumb and two fingers, and then just the thumb and first finger. Having reached proficiency with both hands, take up the same position and suddenly drop to the floor as before, catching the door with one hand as you fall. Constant practice will result in a surprising degree of agility and muscular response, particularly so if the dropping back is done with vigour.

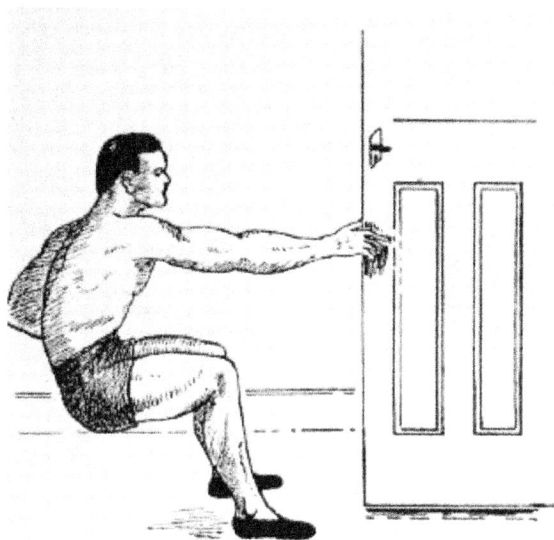

## 8. BENDING A BEER CAP.

Another little stunt that looks very easy, but will surprise you. Procure a cap from the top of a beer or mineral water bottle; the kind that are made of tin with corrugated edges and attempt to bend the outer edges until they meet each other. There are several ways to do this. Place the cap in the gap between the thumb and first finger near the hand, or between the top of the thumb and first finger, or as in the illustration, against the folded finger where the clenched fist makes the task somewhat easier, or simply attempt to crush the beer cap in the palm. Try out all these methods and if you do not succeed with any of them, place the cap between the finger and thumb of the right hand, and bringing the aid of the finger and thumb of the left hand to the job, you should be able to accomplish the feat. Removing the piece of cork usually found in the base of the cap will make the task slightly easier.

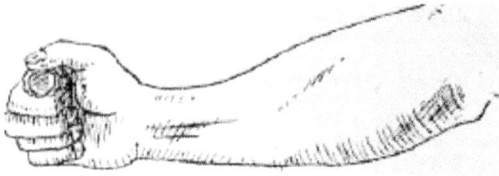

## 9. HANGING FROM A ROPE.

This is a stunt that can be practised in any shed, garage or workshop. Secure a short length of stout rope and tie it securely to a hook in a beam or over a rafter. Stand on a low stool and reaching up as high as possible, grasp the rope with the right hand, all the fingers being close together. Now hang the whole weight of the body on the rope and kick the stool away. Hang on in this position until the arm is thoroughly tired and then repeat with the left hand. This simple feat should on no account be missed where one has the facilities for practising it, for it will develop the entire arm and shoulder muscles and add quite considerably to one's powers of grip. Actually, it is a feat of endurance and therefore no budding strength athlete can afford to miss this opportunity of augmenting his stamina and endurance.

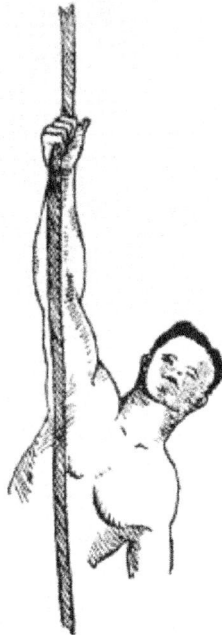

## 10. TEARING A PACK OF CARDS.

One way of tearing the pack is to hold it in the right hand with the palm upwards, thumb round the edges and the right elbow pressed into the side of body for leverage. Take an overhand grip of the top of the pack with the left hand, knuckles upwards, thumb round the opposite edge to the right. Twist the cards one way with the right hand and the other way with the left hand and if your grip is strong enough, they will part in the centre.

Another way is to place both ends of the pack in the palms, the thumbs being pressed against the index fingers of both hands. In this case the thumbs face in the same direction. Now commence the tear with a twisting motion, the right hand twisting inwards and the left hand twisting outwards. Having secured a start, the twist must be kept going until the pack is halved. With this method it is an advantage if the pack rests on the thigh of the right leg, which should be slightly advanced.

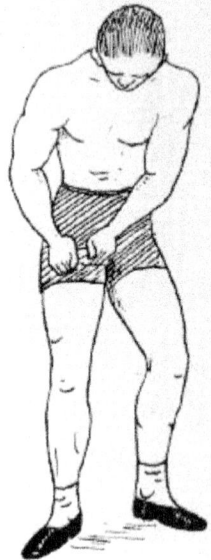

# 11. PRESSING UP FROM THE FLOOR ON FINGER-TIPS.

To develop the grip to its fullest extent, every possible variety of exercise must be utilised, and this one of pressing up from the floor on fingers and thumbs only can be recommended to offset the contractile effect of the usual gripping stunts. Every reader will be familiar with the "Press-up" exercise with the palms of the hands flat on the floor (known in the Services as the " Double Arm Bend and Press,") but few, I imagine, have tried it out on the fingers and thumbs only. It will be advisable for the novice to practice in the ordinary manner with the hands flat on the floor first, before attempting the more advanced style advocated here. Once a certain degree of proficiency is attained, the fingers and thumbs only should be employed. The idea is to spread the fingers to their fullest extent in order to preserve balance.

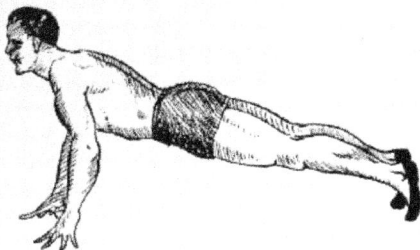

## 12. FINGER LIFTING.

There are two methods of lifting weights with the fingers. One is to lift a light weight off a low bench or stool by the contractile power of the finger tendons. In this case, the weight is held in the middle of the second finger joint and the weight raised by curling the finger up to the hand. The other method employs the tensile strength of the fingers to lift fairly heavy weights from the ground and stand erect with them, the lifting finger being curled into a hook and used as such. All the fingers of both hands should be used in turn, and with practice, one can lift almost as heavy a weight as can be raised with the whole hand. It will be best to use a finger-hook, as illustrated on another page, and even then the fingers will be sore after a few attempts and time must be allowed for them to harden.

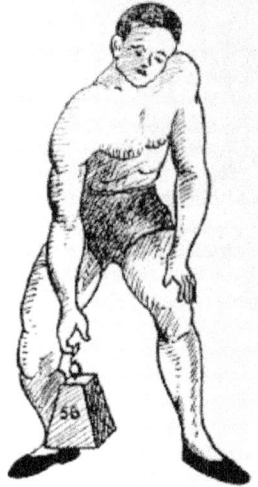

## 13. MAKING A FINGER HOOK.

If you are desirous of approaching anywhere near to the strong man class, it will be advisable for you to make—or have made for you—a finger hook for lifting. As is explained elsewhere in this little book, the contractile strength that can be developed in the fingers is little short of remarkable, and the best way to attain that degree of strength is by the regular use of the finger hook. It is quite easily made from a short length of quarter-inch mild steel, placed in the jaws of a vice and hammered into shape. The loop into which the finger goes is bound with adhesive tape in order to protect the finger. Each finger should be used in turn with gradually increasing weights. With practice, the middle finger should be able to raise within twenty per cent., of that elevated by the entire hand.

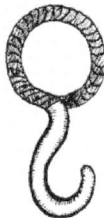

## 14. HOLDING OUT A BROOM WITH FLAT-IRON.

To hold out a heavy bass broom by the further end of the stick is quite a feat of its own for the average man, but as this type of broom is not always available, the ordinary house broom will have td be utilised, and this utensil being of light weight should prove to be well "within one's powers. . To make the feat worth while, a flat-iron may be threaded oh the handle and an attempt made to ascertain one's! strength by the measure of distance the iron is from the hand. Orice this is done, the position should be marked and practice put in by gradually shifting the iron towards the broom end. The grip should be taken near the end of the stick with the knuckles upward, the thumb being well underneath and spread along the handle.

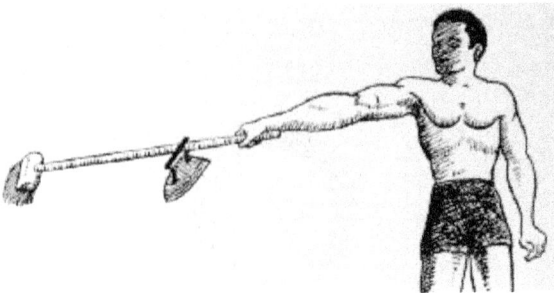

## 15. TEARING A TELEPHONE BOOK.

One way to accomplish this feat is to hold the book with the bound edge resting on the thigh, both hands grasping the leaf edge with the knuckles upwards, back of both hands facing the body. The thumbs should be about two inches apart. Now double the book on itself, causing the leaves to spray and then start the tear by pulling towards the body with the right hand and pushing away with the left hand. Continue to push and pull until the whole of the sprayed pages are started. It will now be an easy matter to complete the halving of the book. This method of starting the tear with a few pages is by far the easiest and although the trick—for trick it really is—may be obvious to many of the audience, speed will come with practice and then the tear will appear so continuous that the book will seem to be halved at one operation.

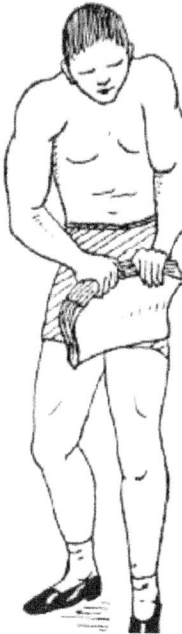

The fairest method is to tear the book from the back—that is, the bound edge—for as it presents a solid edge it becomes a real feat of strength.

## 16. CIRCLING A DUMB-BELL.

This is an exceptionally good exercise for the whole of the wrists. Sit on a chair, with the elbow of the right arm resting on a table, and grasp a round-headed dumb-bell by one end, with the finger* well spaced around the ball. Work the wrist and roll the dumb-bell around in a circle, allowing the further end to describe the fullest possible arc. Revolve the dumb-bell first to the right and then to the left. When the wrist of the right hand begins to tire, change over to the left hand.

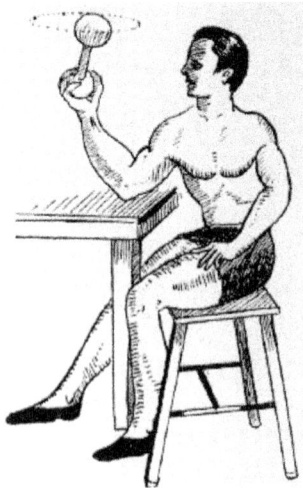

## 17. HOLDING OUT A DISC ON A ROD.

Here is a feat for the bar-bell fans. It consists of holding out a dumb-bell rod on which a disc is held in position by a collar, or collars, and must not be confused with the lift known as the " crucifix " or " muscling out," as it is termed in the States. Place a disc of, say, ten pounds on an eighteen inch rod and secure it in position near the centre with a collar at the rear on both ends. Grasp the rod firmly in the right hand, allowing the little finger to be level with the end of the rod. (In the illustration the grip is taken too far along the bar.) If you can manage the weight, try it out with the left hand, if not, bring the disc in toward the hand a little. Continue to practice as opportunity occurs until the weight can be taken to the far end of the rod. In " muscling out" the strain is on the shoulder and upper arm, but this feat is a real teaser for the forearm and grip.

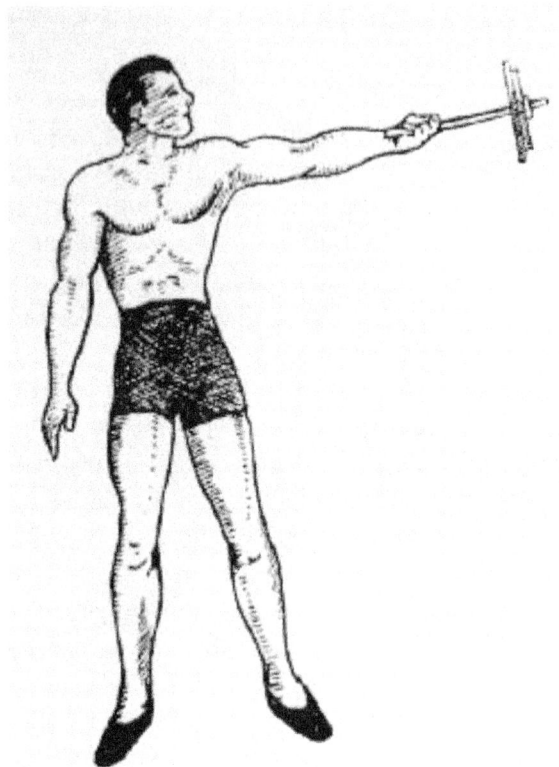

## 18. PICKING UP DISCS.

Here is another feat for the bar-bell fans. It consists of the simple action of picking up a heavy disc by the forceps-like grip of the thumb and fingers. Stand the disc on edge and spreading the thumb well down the sides of the plate, pick it up from the ground and stand erect. These discs are made in various weights, and one should commence with a 25 lb. disc. Secure a good pincer grip and then lift with the shoulder of the arm in use, for you may find that if you attempt to lift the weight by bending the forearm, the discs may escape your hold. Therefore take a grip and stand up, keeping the lifting arm perfectly straight.

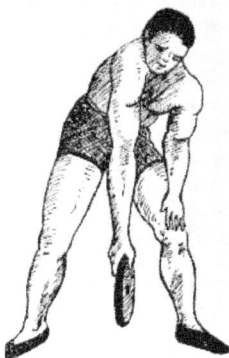

## 19. HOLDING OUT DISCS.

Here is a slight variation on the holding-out feats. The disc is held out at right angles to the body with the plate resting on the spread fingers and kept from toppling over by the pressure of the thumb only. It will be found that the strain is centred on the first and second joints of the fingers and the ball of the thumb. A 10 lb. plate can be used to commence, and you will find that a good deal of practice is necessary before the next size disc can be managed, for the 15 lb. plate has a larger diameter and this means that the strain on the hand is increased out of all proportion to the actual weight. Much will therefore depend on the make of the discs; whether they are of the squat type, or having a wider diameter.

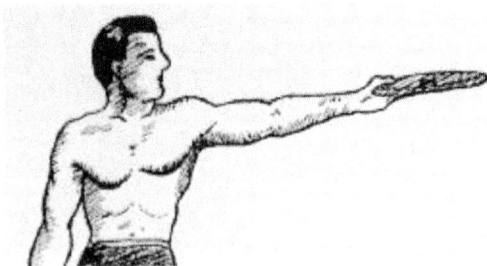

## 20. CIRCLING A BAR-BELL.

This is a rather similar movement to that of winding up a weight, for the muscular action is the same, except that one retains the same grip on the bar all the time. The bar-bell is brought up from the "hang" position, to the front of the body, with the knuckles upwards. It is permissible to dig the elbows into the sides so that the action may be concentrated on the wrjsts and forearms. Keeping the arms rigid, turn the hands upwards and downwards to their fullest extent by wrist action, retaining a full grip on the bar all the time.

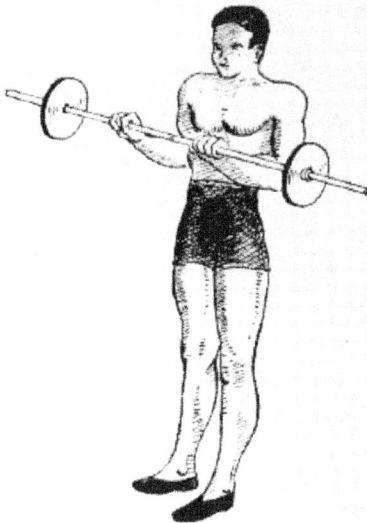

# HOW TO DEVELOP A POWERFUL GRIP

In my considered opinion, a powerful grip is the most important part of the athlete's physical requirements, particularly so in the case of the weight-lifter, and as a weight-lifter myself it is to this sport that I confine my views. In confirmation of this statement I may recall that some years ago, when the "Two Hands Dead Lift" became popular, those contestants whose gripping powers were inadequate to cope with near-record poundages, were permitted by the rules framed by the Weight-Lifters' Association to handle the bar in a reverse grip, which allows the lifter to take hold of the bar with one palm facing the front while the other palm faces the rear. This prevents the bar from rolling off the fingers and naturally makes the lifting of the weight much easier from the gripping angle.

Now I contend that when the grip is fully developed this reverse gripping is unnecessary. As proof of this I may be allowed to instance my attempt, in Paris, to raise a weight of approximately five hundred pounds with a bar of two and a quarter inches diameter. This weight, I was told, had only been lifted by three Frenchmen, all of whom were in the heavy-weight class. I was invited to try it and, much to the surprise of the experts present, I succeeded in doing so at the first attempt, and with both palms facing the same way. The reason for my success, can be explained by the fact that in my training for exhibition lifting, I had for years been exercising with a two and a half inch bar, and this had enormously strengthened my powers of grip. As is now well known, the greater the diameter of the bar one practices with, the stronger becomes the power of the hands and forearm.

There are other methods to develop a steel-like grip which I propose to describe, but to make the subject more interesting to the average reader, I will first of all introduce some of the great figures in Physical Culture history. The man with the most famous grip was undoubtedly Vansittart. He was not a heavy man, but he probably possessed the most phenomenal muscular development ever seen. He carried no spare flesh; consequently his superb muscularity stood out in bold relief, with all the definition of an anatomical chart. And what a grip he possessed. One of his feats was to seize a champagne bottle filled with lead shot, by the neck with one hand, and by manipulating the fingers, slowly work the bottle upwards until the bottom balanced on his palm. Many tried to duplicate this feat, but none succeeded. A fifty-six pound block weight would be lifted by his thumb and forefinger and he could raise two weights of this character, base to base, in the same manner. The tearing of tennis balls into halves was another of his unapproachable feats, and any would-be champion seeking to emulate this, will quickly realise the enormous power required to rend the ball. A further feat consisted of holding out horizontally half a dozen billiard cues between the first and second fingers of one hand; the slender ends being between the fingers. The leverage thus created by the unsupported heavy ends was terrific and may well be imagined. (Apollo, the Scottish Hercules, could perform this feat with five cues.) If the reader fancies his prospects in this direction I would advise him to proceed very carefully, otherwise injury may occur. Naturally, the successful accomplishment of this act was only arrived at by easy stages. First, the empty champagne bottle, then a small quantity of shot to be increased by ounces as progress is made. Again, one billiard cue to commence with; a tennis ball with part of the seams cut, and so on. But Vansittart was a past master of this class of stunt and made a speciality of every feat connected with the power of grip. He was, in fact, billed at the Music Halls as " The Man with the Iron Grip," but whether he could handle heavy weights in the ordinary way, I am unable to say, for he assuredly made no move in the direction of challenging others in pure lifting.

John Gruhn Marks was a German of colossal stature, with a pair of hands the size of small shovels and needless to add, he made good use of them. With this favourable equipment of Nature, his speciality was the lifting of dumbbells with extra thick handles. No competitor was ever able to elevate his pet dumbbells and the reason is simple to explain. First of all he was a heavy-weight and possessed the extra strength natural to that class, then he had long powerful hands and massive forearms with plenty of leverage and finally the advantage of using a unique type of weight. These were solid dumbbells with loose sleeves running over the centre bar. The average lifter attempting to raise the dumbbell would find that the sleeve revolved, because even if he possessed the strength to raise the dumbbell he would fail in getting his hand completely round the thick bar to prevent the sleeve from turning in his hand. Only a man with exceptionally sized hands could duplicate the feat, but Marks had hands that would go completely round the sleeve and moreover by constant practice he had inured his grip to the eccentricities of this novel method of grasping the bar. Part of his performance consisted of breaking horse-shoes with his bare hands, breaking chains by pulling them apart and he would also smash in two with one blow of his fist a chain suspended between two pillars. The links of this chain were of the figure " 8 " type and being very thick, required an enormous output of strength to open them. This old-timer, although favoured by nature, was not content to rest satisfied with the strength inherent in his make-up, but practised progressively from small- handled dumbbells to larger ones; from weak chains to stronger until his hands contained amazing powers of grip and contraction.

A famous name in the annals of strength is that of Thomas Top- ham. He lived long before our time, but his many feats of strength will be remembered for a long while to come. The records show that he was a tall, heavy man, fond of good eating and drinking. While some of the acts he was credited with seem to savour of romance, as for instance his feat of running half a mile with a cask of nails weighing several hundredweights on one shoulder. Others have an air of probability in their favour. One of his claims to fame was a wonderful power of grip and he was wont to display it by crushing a pewter pot in his right hand. It is rumoured that these ale containers were often the cause of wagers between the ale drinkers of that time and Master Topham being a past master of the stunt was often called upon to settle a wager as to whether or no he could crush a particular tankard. What the landlord of the hostelry thought of the business is not on record but he was possibly well compensated for his loss of property. Apropos of this anecdote it may not be out of place to mention that a great grandmother of mine was named Topham and hailed from the same neighbourhood. I have often wondered whether I am a descendant of the original Topham for the coincidence seems strong enough to bear that suspicion, but actually I have never bothered to ascertain.

Samson (Alexandra Zass) the Russian strong man, who will be known to many of my readers, is still displaying his remarkable powers of grip. I have had quite a lot to do with him in one way and another and can vouch for the accuracy of what follows. Samson's special act is in the twisting of chains, unlike Marks, whose method was to pull them apart. There is a reason for this.

The chains used by Samson are of the double loop type, with the ends of the links knotted in the middle. As it is not possible to open the links by a direct pull, Samson gets over the difficulty by first interlocking the links and then by sheer finger strength, bends the loop backward and forwards until it breaks. The broken loop of the link is now in the torm of a hook and can be opened if sufficient pull be exerted on it. Samson does this in quite a novel manner. He connects the chain very tightly around his deflated chest and by tremendous inflation and expansion of the chest, plus extension of the latissimus dorsi muscles, opens the link and sends the chain flying with a loud ping that can be heard all over the Hall. Now, although these anecdotes are concerned with gripping powers only I have had to digress in order to explain the reason why Samson in his act only partly breaks the chain with his hands. He personally considers the preliminary manipulation with the hands to be only a minor part of the act, and that the real feat consists of breaking the chain around the chest. If the reader should be tempted to emulate this feat I would strongly advise him to go slowly and with very light chains, for the breaking of anything—even of string—

over the bare flesh, can be very painful and requires much progressive treatment.

Samson's outstanding powers of grip enable him to perform many very exceptional feats with his hands. Probably the most difficult and one always well received by the audience was the bending of a piece of iron bar usually five-eighths of an inch square, into the shape of a magnet. This I have seen him do with a piece no longer than five inches and believe me, this is some feat, for it permits of little or no leverage to commence the bend. He starts off by holding the bar at the edges with both hands, places the centre on his naked thigh and commences to bend. Once it is out of the straight, he completes the stunt of bringing the two ends of the bar near each other by the sheer gripping power of both hands, and then holding the bar in one hand, closes the ends together. The first part of the act is the bending on the thigh and this can be very painful, so if you are anxious to get into the strong man class, I suggest that you commence with a longer piece of iron, with a smaller diameter and use a leather pad on the thigh. Again, wrapping of the ends with stout canvas gives leverage and saves the hands much soreness. At the same time it is really amazing how quickly one can progress in this direction and develop power in the tendons of the arms and hands. Tolson of Dewsbury is an outstanding proof of this for he succeeded in duplicating this feat of Samson's. Another of the Russian Strong Man's performances was that of lifting by wrist and arm strength a large metal jug. This jug was shaped like a drinking tankard and weighed about sixty pounds. The manner of lifting was to extend the arm across a table and by pure gripping power and wrist strength, to grasp the jug and raise it slowly to a perpendicular position close to one's mouth. Many weightlifters have performed a similar feat to this with a dumbbell, held with the palm well under the bar in order to shorten the leverage. But to raise this novel jug by the handle, with the full weight pulling over and away from the grip is indeed a remarkable feat and requires not only a most powerful grip but exceptional wrist strength and steel-like tendons of the arms. Samson had enormous strength in his thumbs and this was exampled in his business of chain-breaking already mentioned. How much of his strength was inherent and how much was due to cultivation it is difficult to say, but that he must have practised continually is certain, for however much one is favoured by nature in the way of muscular power, it can always be considerably amplified by constant and progressive usage. When one considers that Samson weighs only just over eleven stone, his feats are outstanding.

Brietbart was an American of German extract, and here again his special feats were in the form of tremendous gripping power. Compared with Samson he was a biggish man and a great favourite on the halls. One of his best acts was the tearing in two of a sheet of iron nearly one-eighth of an inch thick. This he achieved in the same manner that one would attempt to tear a pack of cards, an oid and ever popular show of the old-time strong man. (I hope to have something to say of this card-tearing business later.) This sheet of iron measuring roughly six inches square was taken into his hands and torn cleanly in two, and though he challenged all and sundry, no one succeeded in emulating this feat. Speaking as one with some experience, I would say that it would take many months to get anywhere within reach of accomplishment, for long and ardous practice is required, not only for the development of the necessary power of grip, but to get the hands in such a condition that they would be hardened and pickled to withstand the sharp edges of the iron without being damaged. Breitbart evidently commenced by using very thin sheets of metal and as time went on and his powers improved, gradually increased the thickness. It was probably an expensive process, both of time and money, but as a public performer earning hundreds of pounds a week, it certainly proved a good investment.

Caswell, an old opponent of Thomas Inch, was a man around ten and a half stone, who also possessed exceptional gripping powers. At the time that Vansittart was topping the bills of the Music Halls, Caswell was probably the only one to come anywhere within reach of him, and apart from these two, I do not recollect any performer at that time whose powers of grip could be termed phenomenal. Sandow and several others tore packs of cards into halves and quarters, but that was as far as they went in displaying their gripping powers. Caswell was a Londoner by birth and was always very popular for though he never appeared on the stage he could always be relied upon to give a show for charity or any deserving cause. Most of his displays were given at Physical Culture Shows and among the members of the P.C. Clubs he was regarded with awe; so remarkable were his powers of grip. His speciality was the manipulation of fifty-six pound block-weights and ring-weights. He could pick up two block-weights with one hand and perform all manner of tricks with a single one. His fingers were indeed very thick and they were heavily calloused, an absolute necessity this, when one considers the class of act he featured. One of his special feats was to take hold, with thumb and forefinger only, the peg through which the ring of the fifty-six pound weight ran, lift it from the ground and turn it over at shoulder height; then press it aloft. Considering the awkwardness of this stunt and the smallness of the object gripped, it was really spectacular and has seldom or ever been duplicated. The balancing of the weight when inverted, by means of the thumb and forefinger only, to complete the overhead press, was, as can be imagined, extremely difficult. How Caswell obtained his grip strength I do not know, but that it required real hard work to cultivate that degree of ability, I can well understand. He had the reputation of being able to bend pennies with his fingers and even to break them in half, but in my personal opinion it is not possible for any living person to break a penny in half. At least, not a sound and good penny. They have been bent, for I have seen them bent and have bent them myself, but to break one, is, I consider, impossible. When I was still in the doubting stage about its possibilities, I made

47

a test that finally convinced me and that consisted of placing a penny in a vice, gripping the free end with a pair of pliers and employing the full powers of my arms to break the coin. I found that it took thirty movements backwards and forwards before there was any sign at all of its rupture. That test proved to my satisfaction that to break a penny with the hands alone was not possible, but to bend a penny is another matter, for although it requires a certain amount of strength in the fingers, it is somewhat in the nature of a trick. And this is how it is done. Lay the palm of your left hand flat on a table or other flat surface. Now raise all fingers with the exception of the middle one. Place a penny on it well clear of the finger nail, then lower first and third fingers to rest on the outer edges of the coin. Now to actually bend it, you must strike very forcibly and smartly with the clenched fist of the other arm, the two fingers directly over the penny and—this is important—it must be done with full confidence. The blow should be delivered with the heel of the striking hand and directed evenly over the two uppermost fingers. If you are a sedentary worker it will be wise to use a pad, otherwise you may receive injury. And again, if you have slender fingers, it will be well to leave alone. Caswell was also good at holding out the full-sized billiards cues in the manner of Vansittart. I have no information with regard to chain-breaking but he was certainly particularly good at bending stout wire nails. He would completely bend over as many as half a dozen six- inch wire nails held bunched in the hands, and using only one nail, he would interlace it between the fingers of one hand and bend it, by simply closing his fist. Caswell had the quite unusual gift of being as good with the left hand as with the right. In build, Caswell was somewhat average height, whereas Vansittart was a tallish man, so it would appear that the former was better favoured by nature for this class of work than the latter. It is evident that he had no desire to appear on the Music Halls, but had he done so, he would certainly have made a sensation and may have eventually rivalled his contemporary.

The tearing of playing cards was included in the programme of practically every old-time strength performer, and it is fairly safe to say that every one of them claimed to be the real champion of this feat. William Fox, " The miniature Hercules," would show how easily he could tear one pack of cards into halves and then quarters; a performance that always went down well with the public.

Several others' who shall be nameless, claimed to tear one and a half packs; some claimed to tear two packs and all declared the cards to be genuine and untampered with. But the greatest claim of all came from that peerless performer Eugene Sandow, who would perform the feat with THREE packs. Now I have personally attempted card tearing on many occasions but I never succeeded with more than one pack of genuine new cards. Perhaps I did not keep practicing long enough to become expert at it, for it is certainly an expensive method of testing the strength of the hands, but if I had persevered long enough I doubt if I could ever have succeeded with two packs. The strength required to tear one pack is in itself considerable and when some of the performers of that day claimed to be able to tear two or more packs I became credulous and commenced to make inquiries. My investigation eventually yielded fruit for I came across a man who had been attendant to one of the most famous names in the strength game and he told me of how the cards were treated to make easier their resistance to the grip and this is how he explained it. Separate packs of cards were encased at each end in a metal container, leaving exposed only about a quarter of an inch in the dead centre. The packs were then placed in an oven and slowly baked. They were left in the heated oven long enough to thoroughly de-nature the exposed centre portion right through the thickness of the cards, so that when they came to be handled, this centre offered little resistance and being weakened in a straight line down the centre there was no chance of the tear going awry as was the case sometimes with the genuine article. With this method of treatment, two or more packs of the devitalised cards could be torn with little, if any, more strength than that required to rend one genuine pack. And on examination of the packs there was no discolouration or other evidence to show that they had been tampered with. So much for card tearing as a feat of strength. Applied in a straightforward manner it is a very fine exercise to develop the powers of grip, but do not expect to tear more than one pack at a time. Many performers vary this stunt by tearing Telephone books and such volumes into halves. These are no more difficult to handle than playing cards, so long as the principle employed is the same, and here I will explain what that principle is. In order to present a rigid resistance—which is the best one— against one's strength, the grip should be so applied as to allow as little free play to the cards or books as possible. In other words the grip must be close to the centre. Having secured this grip, you must now try to form the cards or book into the shape of the letter " S but only slightly so. This contour effects the rigidity of the object and enables one to push against a more solid resistance. Once you have started the tear, the rest is comparatively easy. Grip firmly and do not allow the cards to slip about. It is quite legitimate to use a little powdered resin between the cards to prevent them slipping. The book being of coarser material will not require this aid.

Thomas Inch was also famed for his powers of gripping and his specialities were dual. He possessed a thick handled dumbbell—in fact, he had two—which he challenged all comers to lift and he had also a grip machine of the nut-cracker type. Many of my readers, will remember that Len Harvey the boxer, conquered the latter and achieved a certain amount of fame in doing so. But allow me first of all to deal with the dumbbells. One weighed one hundred and thirty pounds and the other one hundred and eighty. The diameter of the handle of each was about two and a quarter inches and unlike the sleeve used by Marks it was fixed and not loose. The handle was hollow and had in its centre a hole of about a quarter of an inch diameter, but what this was for no one discovered. The dumbbell was evenly balanced and was quite nice to handle, provided that one had suitable hands. To lift a thick-handled, heavy dumbbell one must not only have long hands but they must be fairly soft. A man used to hard manual labour, with the calloused hands that this type of work induces would have little chance of elevating this type of bar. He might be able to grip the bar, but he would not lift it. For this reason. To be able to exert full power, one has to apply as great a surface of the fingers and thumb to the bar as possible. If the hands happen to be hard and knobbly, there will be gaps in the surface applied to the bar and consequently the clinging effect is reduced. Other things being equal, the sendentary worker is best suited to the accomplishment of a feat of this kind. Now, the grip machine mentioned before, was to my mind, a more effective method of essaying one's gripping powers and a fairer test. As I have said, the appliance was of the nut-cracker type, that is to say, a length of steel coiled once or twice in the centre with the ends brought to face each other. The test was to grip the ends hard enough so that they would meet. I have seen Inch do this and although I have attempted the feat I could never succeed in getting the last eighth of an inch. These gripping stunts, like all the others in the category of the strong man's bags of tricks, require long and constant practice, and I was busy, always attempting to excel at my own feats, for as I am a firm believer in originality I isought for other fields to conquer. My pet gripping stunt was known as the Grip Tug-O-War. I invented it for purely demonstration purposes and it was acclaimed as sensational, though personally I did not think that there was a great deal in it. Let me explain first of all how it worked. I had a pair of iron loops specially made in the form of triangles. Attached to one corner of each loop was a stoutish rope. Eight men were asked to come upon the stage and I assembled them four on each side to take part in the tug-o-war. I placed the two triangles firmly in my right hand with the sides running parallel and the men took hold of the ropes. Now if the men pulled in opposite directions and their combined strength proved stronger than my grip, the two triangles would separate and my hand would be opened. But the power of grip I possessed for this particular trick proved to be very great; so much so that it withstood the power of the eight men. The secret was in the way that the two pieces of iron were held. One of the triangles was resisted by means of the base of the thumb and held partly across the palm. So long as I held the other loop in my hand it could not escape, the other triangle loop being held in the crook of my fingers. The paralleled handles were not held closely but about two inches apart. It was the curl of the fingers that took most of the strain and as all strength fans are well aware, the power of resistance in this manner is very great. It was not actually a feat of grip, but rather one of resisting the opening of the hand, for I had worked it out that way. I knew that the ligaments of the fingers possessed great contractile power and provided that I exerted sufficient strength to keep the fingers crooked, it would require great force to extend them outwards. So long as I held one triangle in my fingers, the other triangle would be assisting in its own peculiar way. What gave me the idea of this stunt was an event that happened in Aberdeen, where Samson was appearing at one Music Hall and I at another. I went along to pay him a visit and he introduced me to his pet monkey, an animal weighing about thirty pounds only, but like his master, exceptionally strong. The monkey extended his hand through the bars of his cage and not wishing to be unsocial I accepted his gesture of friendship. But to my surprise, the ape grasped my fingers tightly and gave such a tremendous tug that I had to exert all my strength to prevent being pulled into the cage. The power in that monkey's paw was terrific. The incident passed off but it set me wondering where all that force came from. There is no doubt that constant hanging by the hands from branches of trees in their wild state and from the bars of their cage in captivity has developed enormous tensile strength in their fingers. It is evident, that weight for weight, their hands are probably stronger than ours, but I doubt if they could grip as much as the average manual worker in a test such as that furnished by a grip machine, for their major power lies in the finger tendons. However, it was this principle of finger strength that I applied to my grip tug-o-war stunt and it was certainly a success.

On one occasion, when I was staying at Wimbledon before the last war, my gripping powers came in useful to relieve a man suffering from toothache, and this person, strangely enough, was a dentist by profession. He came to me in great pain and said that he had visited all the local dentists, but none could manage to extract the aching tooth. It was a great molar and firmly embedded in the lower jaw bone. He had brought the appropriate forceps with him and said quite frankly that he did not care a hang how amateurish my efforts, so long as the offending tooth came out, for he had fortified himself with several stiff doses of brandy. I had a go and managed to get the thing out at the first attempt and his relief and gratitude was so great that he offered to train me without fee or charge to become a dentist. But, being busy in my own line, I had to decline with thanks.

Have you ever tried to crush an egg endways up between the hands? It is a favourite stunt and the idea is to place the egg between the palms lengthwise and then pressing inward to attempt to break it. It is not possible to do this under these conditions for the structure of the egg is such that it resists all pressure. However, when this trick was last suggested to me, I proposed something better. I said that I would not only crush the egg, but accomplish this with one hand. I did so, but if I had abided by the rules and held the egg properly I should have failed. But, actually I took a slightly different grip and squeezed; with the result that we had egg all over the place, on nly clothes and those of the bystanders. Luckily, it cannot be done fairly, for it is a messy job.

I have often marvelled that weight-lifters, as a rule, do not pay more attention to the grip. There appears to be no limitation to the height to which the fully developed grip of the human hands could be trained, and its full potentialities must be enormous. I am fully convinced that at least another twenty per cent, could be added to the poundage of some of the lifts if the lifter's grip was more carefully cultivated. Take any lift of a heavy poundage and you will find lifters who are able to " jerk " more than they can " clean." This should not be so. I was addicted to this failure myself, through not sufficiently cultivating my extreme possibilities of grip power. I could jerk three hundred and thirteen pounds but was only able to clean two hundred and eighty pounds. Of course, I can excuse myself now and say that this was a long time ago, but I should have known better. Any lifter should be able to clean a weight up to jerking possibilities and the failure to do so is only insufficient gripping powers, for the other muscles are strong enough to accomplish the lift. In the " two hands snatch " we have a lift capable of a very high poundage, but the lifter often fails to record his best owing to lack of grip.

As an observer of athletics to-day, instead of an active participant, I can see how success can be greatly advanced by means of developing one's powers of grip to its absolute maximum. My advice to all would-be champions is, make sure that you develop a powerful grip.

## THE FOREARMS OF FAMOUS STRONG MEN COMPARED

The forearm is not an easy part of the body to develop, for the simple reason that the muscle fibres are closely packed and with little flesh between. Like the calf muscles, they are in continual use and therefore, real hard work is indicated in order to develop them to any size. But the effort is well worth while for a well-rounded forearm with a shapely wrist is a real asset of masculine beauty, besides which, a considerable increase in strength of the grip will be noted before ever any alteration of size is registered. This is due to the number of tendons, and as is well known, the tendons are considerably stronger than muscular structure.

To give the reader some idea of the development possibilities of this part, I am including the forearm measurements of some Famous Strong Men.

| | Forearm ins. | Height ft. | Height ins. |
|---|---|---|---|
| APOLLON (France) ... ... ... | 18¼ | 6 | 0½ |
| APOLLON, YOUNG (Tolson) ... ... | 14½ | 5 | 6 |
| CASWELL, W. P. ... ... ... | 13½ | 5 | 4½ |
| DARIAZ, MAURICE ... ... ... | 13¼ | 5 | 4½ |
| ELLIOTT, LAUNCESTON ... ... | 15½ | 6 | 1½ |
| GORNER, HERMAN ... ... ... | 16½ | (over | 6ft.) |
| HACKENSCHMIDT, GEORGES ... | 15½ | 5 | 8 |
| INCH, THOMAS ... ... ... | 14¾ | 5 | 10½ |
| MASSIMO, CLEVIO ... ... ... | 15 | 5 | 8½ |
| MEAD, ALAN P. ... ... ... | 13½ | 6 | 1 |
| SANDOW, EUGENE ... ... ... | 16½ | 5 | 8½ |
| SAXON, ARTHUR ... ... ... | 14¾ | 5 | 10 |
| WALKER, RONALD ... ... ... | 14¾ | 5 | 10¾ |
| WOOD, HAROLD ... ... ... | 14½ | 5 | 11¾ |
| VANSITTART, CHARLES ... ... | 14½ | 5 | 9 |

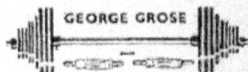
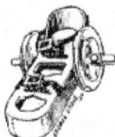
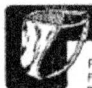
62

.

Printed in Great Britain
by Amazon